CAREERS IN
GERIATRIC NURSING

NURSES CARING FOR THE RAPIDLY EXPANDING ELDERLY POPULATION

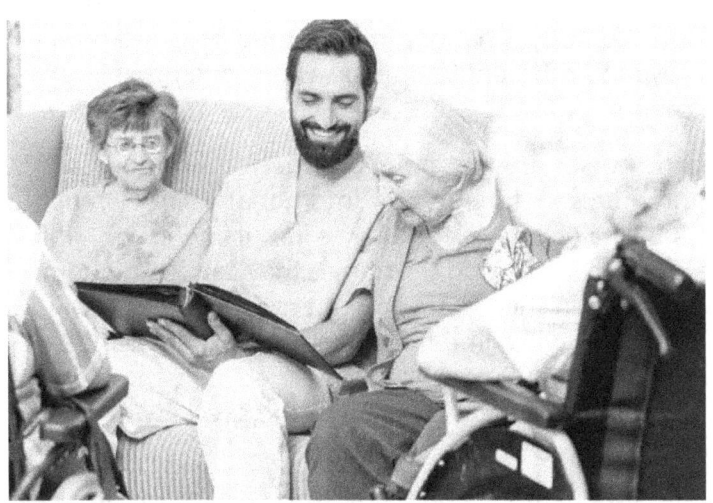

GERIATRIC NURSES SPECIALIZE IN CARING for elderly adults. As most people get older, their bodies and minds start to slow down and wear out. Their immune systems weaken along with their bones and they become more vulnerable to disease and accidents. Because of this, elderly people typically need more medical care than younger people. Most of their care is provided by geriatric nurses, which makes these professionals highly valued by those people who depend on them. In addition to preventing health emergencies, geriatric nurses have a huge impact on the quality of life for both patients and their families.

Caring for older adults is both challenging and rewarding. The work requires knowledge in all areas of healthcare, and a willingness to keep up with the expanding scientific base for geriatric medicine. There is much we do not yet know about aging, but we do know that it is complex, involving biological, psychological, and social changes. We also know that elderly individuals are different than other adults. They need special care, since a minor health problem like the flu or a fall can spin out of control quickly. Changes in their metabolism can mean they respond differently to medications and other treatments.

Geriatric nurses are first trained to perform traditional nursing duties. Before getting into geriatrics, they must earn a Bachelor of Science degree in nursing (BSN), which takes four years. During that time, they can learn about geriatric care in the classroom, but most of what they need to know will come from hands-on experience. After getting at least 200 hours of that experience, they can sit for an exam to become certified in the specialty of geriatrics.

The job outlook for trained geriatric nurses is excellent and getting better every day. The US is experiencing a so-called "Silver Tsunami" as the population ages faster than any other time in history. The fastest-growing age group is over 80, and with Baby Boomers now entering their 60s, the demand for geriatric care is outpacing the supply of trained professionals. This is great news for aspiring geriatric nurses. Consider that people who are 65 or older account for one-half of all hospital admissions, yet just one percent of registered nurses and only three percent of advanced practice registered nurses are certified in geriatrics. There is definitely a demand for more professionals in this healthcare specialty!

Opportunities are everywhere because people everywhere get older. Geriatric nurses will find that jobs are plentiful in long-term care facilities (nursing homes), assisted living facilities, outpatient clinics, hospitals, rehabilitation centers, senior care centers, retirement centers, and hospice settings. There are also home healthcare agencies that arrange for nursing care in elderly people's homes.

Geriatric nurses enjoy good pay and flexibility. They have the choice of working for a single employer or rotating through different settings assigned by an agency. For the nurse who likes to be on the move, traveling nurses are in demand. It is a great way to see the country and get paid considerably more than a staff nurse.

WHAT YOU CAN DO NOW

START LAYING THE FOUNDATION FOR your future career in geriatric nursing while in high school. Start by making sure you are on a college track. College admission requirements vary, but most nursing programs require four years of math and science. There is plenty of competition for these programs. To get a leg up, take as many Advanced Placement (AP) classes as possible and keep your GPA high.

Talk to your high school counselor about taking the College Level Examination Program (CLEP) tests. If you are good at taking tests or are especially advanced in some subjects, CLEP tests can give you a head start on your college program. There are 33 different subjects that are eligible for college credits if you pass the CLEP tests.

Outside of school, you can get a head start by taking classes in CPR and first aid. These classes will be required in nursing school, so why not get them out of the way now?

Get some real world experience in geriatric nursing by volunteering at a nursing home or senior center. Some hospitals offer summer volunteer programs for high school students. You can ask to be assigned to the geriatric department. Volunteering can give you a good idea of what to expect in this career, plus it will add to the weight of your nursing school application.

Consider joining HOSA-Future Health Professionals if it is available at your school. This international student organization is recognized by the US Department of Education and the Health Science Education Division of ACTE (Association for Career and Technical Education). Its mission is to promote career opportunities in the healthcare industry and provide encouragement to all health science students.

HISTORY OF THE CAREER

GERIATRIC NURSING, AS A SPECIALIZED PROFESSION in the US, is relatively new. While the profession is less than 70 years old, the need to care for people in their declining years has been recognized since ancient times. For example, Egyptian hieroglyphs (circa 2800 BC) portray a person bent with age, leaning on a staff for support. It is perhaps the oldest illustration representing the damaging effects of osteoporosis, a disease that has long been the bane of the aged. Descriptions of afflictions caused by aging continued in Egypt through the written word. In 1550 BC, the oldest and most important medical papyri of ancient Egypt suggested that the primary cause of physical decline in old age was heart disease.

A series of serious writings about the aging processes were published in the 19th century. Most notable was the series of articles by early American physician Benjamin Rush. *On the Condition of the Body and Mind in Old Age* and *Remarks on the Diseases of Old People,* were published in 1805. Welsh physician, George Edward Day, wrote the first entire book on the subject in 1848. He offered the physician's perspective on a number of ills of the aged, and expressed dissatisfaction with the way other physicians dismissed the special needs of elderly patients.

It was also in the 1800s that renowned nurse, Florence Nightingale, set about improving the care of older people in the hospital setting. She became the first person to become a geriatric nurse and eventually helped develop the nursing home concept in England. The first nursing homes in the US were also established in the mid-19th century. They were primarily charitable institutions run by religious organizations. They were only partially successful in meeting the need for nursing care. Many elderly people of the day were housed in poor houses or rural poor farms.

The word "geriatrics" was first used near the end of the 19th century. Dr. Ignatz Leo Nascher of Austria coined the term by writing a number of articles on geriatrics, followed by a book entitled, Geriatrics: The Diseases of Old Age and Their Treatment.

Modern Geriatric Nursing

The specialty of geriatric nursing emerged in the 1950s with the publication of the first geriatric nursing textbook. The field was pioneered by a number of nurses, including Doreen Norton. Norton was widely respected for devoting her life to improving the care of aging people. She conducted research on previously neglected problems, designed management tools that are still used today, and established which equipment should be required on geriatric wards. She lectured tirelessly and her publications attracted worldwide acclamation.

The number of nursing homes in the US surged when the federal government offered matching funds to nursing home vendors in 1950, but the quality of care did not keep up with the quantity. When Medicare/ Medicaid was enacted in 1965, the number of nursing home beds doubled, and after calls for tougher regulations by President Nixon, the quality of geriatric care began to rise.

Most direct care for older persons is provided by nurses. The first geriatric nursing standards were published in 1968, an event that led to the certification of geriatric nurses. The first professional group for the geriatric specialty was formed within the American Nurses Association in the late 1960s. Standards of practice for geriatric nursing were published by that group. The first professional association devoted entirely to geriatric nursing, the National Gerontological Nursing Association, was founded in 1984.

Geriatric nursing care was pioneered primarily by women. The exception was Dr. Les Libow, who created the first fellowship in geriatric medicine at City Hospital Center (Mt. Sinai). He is also recognized for introducing resident rotations in geriatrics and started a teaching nursing home in 1967.

The Veterans Administration (VA) has been a major influence in the development of geriatric care in the U.S. The 1970s saw a significant increase in aging veterans. Leaders at the VA noted its potential effects on the main healthcare system available to veterans. The Geriatrics and Extended Care Services (GEC) was created to provide help for veterans with chronic conditions, life-limiting illnesses, frailty, or disability associated with aging. The VA also developed numerous teaching nursing homes.

The National Academy of Medicine, formerly called the Institute of Medicine, issued a report entitled *Improving Quality of Care in Nursing Homes* in 1986. It detailed independent research into the quality of care and quality of life in long-term care, including nursing homes, home health agencies, residential care facilities, and even family-based care. It identified problem areas and offered recommendations that caught the attention of federal and state policymakers. The result was a variety of nursing home regulations being tacked on to the Office of Budget Reconciliation Act (OBRA) in 1987. Among them was the need for physician services, nursing aide training, restraint and psychotropic drug reduction, and guidelines on reducing polypharmacy (the simultaneous use of multiple drugs to treat a single ailment or condition).

The geriatric nursing specialty has advanced significantly in recent years, mostly through advancing education initiatives. Large-scale education initiatives have been funded by various foundations associated with leading teaching hospitals. Independent groups like the Geriatric Nursing Education Consortium have created more effective teaching tools and provided improved content in geriatric nursing education programs. The American Association of Colleges of Nursing along with the Hartford Institute for Geriatric Nursing established bachelor degree curricular guidelines for geriatric nursing care programs.

WHERE YOU WILL WORK

AMERICANS ARE LIVING LONGER THAN EVER. In the 1950s, when geriatric nursing was taking shape as a specialty, the average lifespan was about 10 years shorter than it is today. At that time, the majority of elderly people were cared for in nursing homes, but along with the increasing average life span, many other things have changed. Nursing homes are no longer the primary employer of geriatric nurses. Consider this: about 13 percent of the population is over the age of 65, but only 4 percent of them live in nursing homes. This means geriatric nurses can be found working in a variety of settings.

Geriatric nurses are often employed at healthcare facilities such as hospitals and outpatient clinics. In hospitals, they may be assigned to the geriatric unit. However, it is more likely they will be working with treatment teams that have large older patient populations, such as outpatient surgery, cardiology, rehabilitation, ophthalmology, and dermatology.

A growing area is geriatric mental health, where geriatric nurses help care for older patients with psychiatric conditions, such as depression, anxiety, Alzheimer's, and age-related dementia. The conditions of the health of patients determine what type of facility they reside in, but most will be in healthcare settings outside of nursing homes.

Other common practice settings include rehabilitation facilities, retirement communities, senior centers, community health agencies, assisted living facilities, hospice settings, and generally anywhere elderly people reside. The services provided depend on each particular patient's health conditions. Only patients in nursing homes require 24/7 skilled nursing care.

Some geriatric nurses also work in home healthcare, traveling to patients' homes to care for them there.

Geriatric nurses have the choice of working for a single employer or rotating through different settings assigned by an agency.

THE WORK YOU WILL DO

GERIATRIC NURSES HELP CARE FOR PEOPLE over the age of 50. They generally care for medical needs, provide hygiene assistance, conduct routine physical and mental health assessments, and help with treatments that usually become necessary after a certain age. Geriatric nurses are skilled in multiple facets of elderly patient care, from treatment planning to rehabilitation and mental health and social connectivity. Their primary goal is to protect the mental and physical health of their patients so that they can remain independent and active as long as possible.

The health needs of older people are uniquely challenging. As we age, our bones and immune system weaken, making us more susceptible to traumatic falls and debilitating illnesses. Metabolism changes with aging, adding to the complexity of health needs. A younger person can break a leg skiing and be back on the slopes in a couple of months. An older person does not bounce back so easily. In fact, a broken hip can lead to a serious disability or even death. Likewise, the flu is a miserable inconvenience for most people, but those over the age of 65 are at a much higher risk of developing complications that require hospitalization. It is estimated that 85 percent of flu deaths occur in this age range.

Chronic health conditions are also more likely to afflict older adults. It is not unusual for an elderly person to have multiple conditions, such as cancer, arthritis, diabetes, hearing impairment, cardiovascular disease, or failing eyesight. In addition to these physical problems, they often have cognitive difficulties that can create additional challenges for the geriatric nurse. Various forms of age-related dementia like Alzheimer's disease affect memory, thinking ability, and confusion. Patients with cognitive problems may be disoriented and uncooperative, or downright angry and mean. They may forget to take necessary medications or refuse to eat or get out of bed. Geriatric nurses are able to remain patient and compassionate when dealing with those who are unintentionally difficult.

In addition to treatment, prevention is an important part of geriatric nursing. These professionals are trained to watch vigilantly for any signs of emerging medical conditions. They monitor patients who are bedridden, inspect homes for possible safety problems, and watch over people in retirement centers and nursing homes. They educate elderly people and their families on how to best prevent illness and accidents.

Geriatric nurses have multiple responsibilities, but a typical day might require them to do the following:

- Assess patient's mental health and cognitive skills

- Review and recognize patients' immediate and chronic health problems

- Organize and administer prescribed medications

- Measure and record vital signs

- Help patients complete prescribed exercise routines

- Connect patients with local resources as needed
- Help with patients' daily needs like bathing, dressing, and using the bathroom
- Transport patients to doctor's visits
- Watch for signs of elder abuse

Hospital Care

A geriatric nurse's specific duties will vary somewhat depending on the environment. For example, in a hospital setting, geriatric nurses work as part of a team under the direction of a doctor. They are usually assigned to a department that treats a high number of older patients, such as outpatient surgery, rehabilitation, cardiology, ophthalmology, dermatology, and geriatric mental health. Therefore, nurses might see patients who have suffered heart attacks, been injured in a fall, or are demonstrating signs of dementia such as Alzheimer's disease. The geriatric nurse would assist a doctor with patient examinations or during surgical procedures or other treatments. In this setting, the geriatric nurse might also perform blood tests, administer medications, and conduct preliminary observations to determine mental status.

Patients are only hospitalized long enough to have surgery, be treated for immediate acute injuries, or be diagnosed. Once initial treatment and/or diagnosis is completed, plans are arranged for any necessary ongoing care elsewhere.

Long-Term Care

In a long-term care (LTC) facility, elderly patients are called "residents" since that is where they live. Instead of working briefly with a person in a hospital, geriatric nurses provide ongoing care for a long period of time, which often means until the end of life. In this setting, the nurses become the residents' primary caregiver. As a result, they become very familiar with each person's condition, and are the first to observe any changes in condition and respond accordingly.

Long-term care usually involves some type of therapy, such as range-of-motion exercises, therapeutic massage, or respiratory therapy. Other LTC duties may include dressing wounds, assisting with adaptive equipment, working with ventilators and catheters, and taking care of tube feedings. Unlike the hospital setting, geriatric nurses in LTCs are not directly supervised.

Healthcare Advocate

The geriatric nurse is first and foremost a caregiver like any other kind of nurse. However, due to the special issues involved with geriatrics, they are also called upon to be advocates, educators, and case managers for their patients.

As healthcare advocates, geriatric nurses provide myriad services for their elderly patients. They may translate medical jargon, act as a spokesperson for the patient, and help calm fears. They also consult with patients and their families to evaluate treatment options. They help them prioritize their options, determine what treatments are actually necessary, and decide what is most important to them. One of the biggest concerns elderly patients have in common is insurance. Insurance can be confusing, especially when transitioning upon retirement. Geriatric nurses have taken on the responsibility of guiding patients through their coverage and helping them find answers to the questions that inevitably arise.

Nurse Educator

Educating patients and their families is a big part of the geriatric nurse's job. A person goes through all kinds of changes during the aging process and along the way, many questions arise. Geriatric nurses can help explain what to expect and how to deal with common health concerns like incontinence, falls from loss of balance, changing sleeping and eating patterns, and sexual issues. They offer advice about preventing disease and injury, as well as how to adjust to necessary lifestyle changes. They teach loved ones how to care for patients with certain medical conditions at home. They explain the patient's medication regimen and recommend ways to ensure compliance.

Certified Case Manager

Some geriatric nurses become certified case managers after gaining experience in a LTC or in home care. It is an autonomous position, with additional responsibilities such as working with new admissions, assessing patient conditions, and developing individualized care plans. LTC residents and home care patients do not require hospitalization, but most do have health issues that require medication, dietary changes, daily exercise routines, and sometimes special equipment such as walkers or blood sugar monitors. Geriatric case manager nurses help design these plans, evaluate and update them as needed, and teach patients and their families how to follow the care plans. They also act as a liaison between patients, their families, healthcare providers, and community resources. Case managers sometimes also provide nursing care for their patients.

Geriatric Nursing Assistant (CNA)

Like all forms of nursing, geriatric care requires teamwork. One member of the team is the geriatric nursing assistant (CNA), sometimes known as a geriatric aide, depending on the environment. Geriatric CNAs help care for elderly people in hospitals, nursing homes, private homes, and adult daycare centers. Their primary responsibility is to help with personal care, such as dressing, grooming, bathing, feeding, and toileting. In the case of home care, they may also provide some light housekeeping like doing laundry or preparing meals. They may also perform basic nursing tasks like checking blood pressure, administering medications, or helping with exercise regimens.

Geriatric Nurse Practitioner

The most highly educated and skilled member of the team is the geriatric nurse practitioner. These professionals can do many of the same tasks as a doctor. In a hospital or clinic, they often perform initial patient evaluations, conduct diagnostic tests, and prescribe medications, without direction from a doctor. Geriatric nurse practitioners often specialize in caring for people with specific conditions like cancer, osteoporosis, broken bones, or terminal illnesses. Having extensive knowledge of a certain health issue allows them to provide the best possible care. When loved ones have concerns, the practitioner can provide expert counseling to help them cope with difficult circumstances. Geriatric nurse practitioners who work in LTCs or home healthcare settings are in a position of authority. They have the final say in the care and management of patients and typically supervise other nurses.

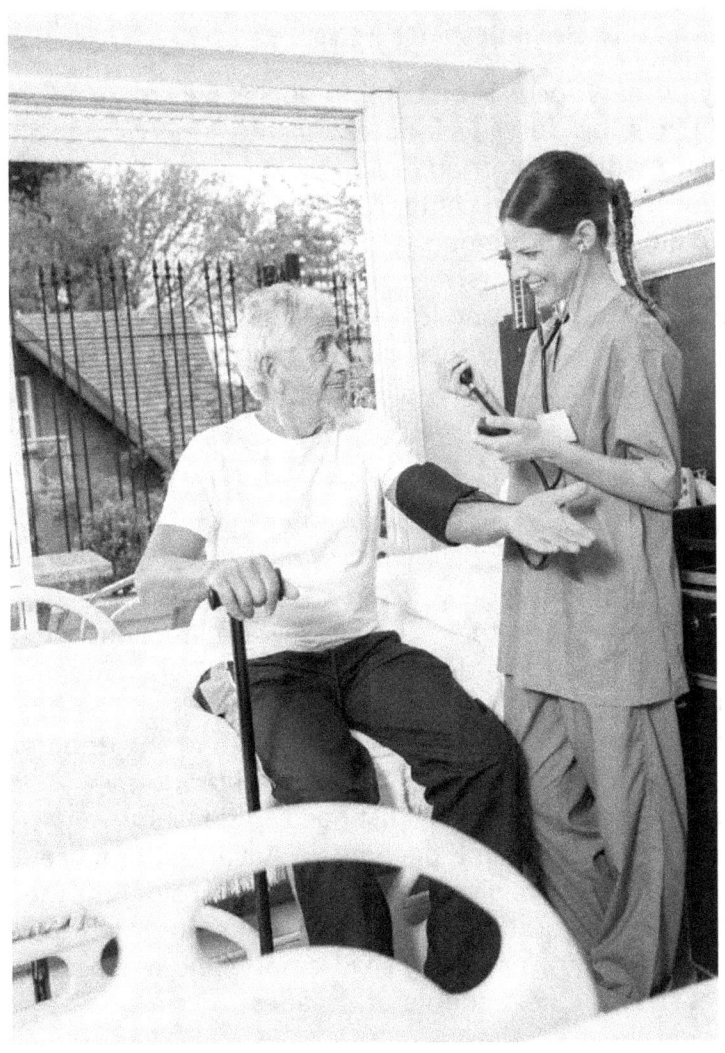

STORIES OF GERIATRIC NURSES

I Am a Professional Coach for Nurses

"My primary focus is on helping nurses overcome what I call 'mission drift.' As a nurse training supervisor at an urban medical center and later while managing a senior rehabilitation center, I noticed a common problem among the nurses. They all started out with passion and pure intentions, but over time they were buried in the work and lost sight of the possibilities. My job is to redefine their goals, remind them of why they chose nursing, and help them realize their potential.

For nurses, the field of geriatrics has more opportunities for career advancement than any other specialty I can think of. There is a nurse shortage in general, but in the geriatric arena, the gap is huge. Now consider that there are very few geriatricians and the number is going down every year. Ask any older adult who takes care of them and they will tell you it is a nurse, not a doctor. To me, that says that the door is wide open for nurses who want more autonomy, money, and respect. They just need to get some additional training and become an Advanced Practice Nurse (APRN) specializing in geriatrics. Considering the size of the older adult population, I estimate there is a need for 10 times as many APRNs now, and maybe 20 times over the next couple of decades.

Another great area for geriatric nurses to consider is

research. An advanced education is needed, but what an exciting future there is for nurse researchers in this field. Grants, especially from NIH, are plentiful due to the pressing need to understand more about the aging process and how nurses can provide the most effective care. This is the kind of work that could elevate a geriatric nurse's career and bring back the excitement felt when first entering the profession."

I Work at a Senior Health Center

"I have a lot of responsibilities so my days are fast-paced. I perform walk-in triage, review lab results, coordinate hospital admissions and ER transfers, supervise nursing assistants, and complete tons of paperwork. Then there are the usual nursing tasks like blood draws, administering medications, catheter insertions, and IV hydration.

This facility provides continuity of care from inpatient to outpatient. I used to worry about patients going home, being isolated, maybe disabled, but technology has fixed that problem here. We now issue iPads to our more vulnerable transitioning patients who are being discharged. The tablets are used to conduct electronic visits with a nurse at regular intervals. It's not as good as having a home-care nurse, but it has proven to reduce readmissions significantly. Using the tablet, I'm able to perform a visual exam and see if there are any signs of distress, listen to breathing and check heart rate, monitor any changes in condition, discuss medications, and make sure discharge instructions are followed.

I love working with elderly people. Most are sweet and funny. Difficult patients do come along, but my job is to reassure them and give them the care they need. It is very satisfying to see an older patient recover from illness and be able to résumé a normal life.

My advice to future geriatric nurses is to never stop learning. Attend seminars and lectures, and take advantage of online learning opportunities. The scientific knowledge of aging is expanding every day. You need to keep up to provide the best possible care. Also, consider learning a second language. There is a tremendous shortage of nurses who can communicate with elderly patients in their native languages. Being able to speak to them would make you invaluable."

PERSONAL QUALIFICATIONS

CARING FOR THE ELDERLY IS A REWARDING, yet challenging career choice. Working with aging patients is more complex than it might seem on the surface. Starting at about age 50, people start to experience all kinds of physiological, cognitive, and emotional changes. There are social changes, too, that complicate life as we get older. Having knowledge in all areas of healthcare and keeping up with the advancing science for geriatric medicine are a challenge, but it takes more than knowledge to be a good geriatric nurse.

It takes a special type of person to work in geriatrics. At the very least, you must enjoy being around elderly people. It can be a joy, but you must be prepared to be frustrated or disheartened at times. People are individuals and the aging process will affect each one differently. Some will take things in stride and may even be cheerful.

Others might be sad, frightened, or cranky because their health is failing and/or they are in pain. You will need to be very patient, understanding, and especially observant in order to know what kind of care is needed.

Compassion is vital when looking after aging patients. By the time most geriatric patients need nursing care, they are near the end of life. Some may be ready for hospice care, but usually it is a matter of medical issues that are starting to pile up and accelerate. They do not need, and usually do not want, your sympathy. They do need and deserve compassion. They are likely to become incontinent or unable to bathe themselves, which is understandably embarrassing and a blow to personal pride. It is not unusual for people in this position to be grumpy about needing someone else to take care of these basic needs. The best way to approach them is with compassion and understanding.

Having empathy is good, but you must keep it in check. This can be difficult when you are developing close relationships with the people in your constant care. Every day you will be dealing with human suffering, emergencies, and other stresses. It takes emotional strength and stability to handle the ups and downs, and especially the inevitable depressing events like the death of a patient.

Patience is a virtue for all nurses, but particularly so for those working in geriatrics. Elderly patients may speak slowly or be easily confused. Some can be easily irritated and difficult. It takes patience to listen carefully and let emotional flares subside. Patience is also needed to deal with family members who may have conflicting feelings about someone outside the family caring for their loved one.

Communications skills are key. Geriatric nurses must be able to slow down and listen carefully. They need to clearly explain instructions, such as how and when to take medication or how to use assistive devices. They must be able to effectively relate the patient's needs to the other health professionals on the team. They also communicate with family members, which is not always easy when balancing patient needs and desires with the demands of family, which may differ.

You must always be ready to slow down and listen carefully. Geriatric nurses are responsible for many details. For starters, they have to make sure their patients get the correct treatments and take the prescribed doses of medicines at the right times. Just as important is watching for signs of potential problems. Older patients are at a high risk of developing serious medical conditions such as cancer, stroke, heart disease, Alzheimer's disease, and osteoporosis. It is vital that the geriatric nurse be observant and check each patient's medical chart diligently to prevent potential emergencies.

Geriatric nurses typically work with multiple patients, each with multiple health needs. Since no two patients are alike, it takes excellent organizational skills to ensure that each patient is given appropriate care according to their individual needs.

ATTRACTIVE FEATURES

WORKING WITH THE ELDERLY PROVIDES many intangible rewards that you will not discover in any other healthcare sector. Patients and their families deeply appreciate geriatric nurses because they have such a positive impact on their quality of life. Everyone wants to stay independent as long as possible while feeling better physically, mentally, and emotionally. That is the ultimate goal of the geriatric nurse. Add tangible rewards like good pay, benefits, and flexible schedules and it is easy to understand why geriatric nurses are happy in their careers.

Geriatrics is bursting at the seams. The elderly population is soaring in the US, and by 2040, the government expects that more than a fifth of the population will be over the age of 65. About 1.3 million seniors live in nursing homes now and long waiting lists already exist at many facilities. Even more senior citizens require regular medical treatment and care, and seek it out elsewhere. All this means is geriatric nurses are in high demand. Employment experts predict job growth to be much faster than that in other occupations. When choosing a career in geriatric nursing, you can expect to be working in a field with solid job prospects and unequaled job security. Plus, you can pick and choose where and how much you want to work.

Geriatric nurses have the opportunity to make a real difference in someone's life. Elderly patients truly need the services they provide. You may literally be the one who keeps them breathing, nourished, clean, and functional. Nobody wants to become helpless or less than fully capable of caring for themselves, but that is the reality that often comes with aging. Geriatric nursing is on the front line of caregiving, making the final years the best they can possibly be. What could be more professionally and personally satisfying than that?

In most geriatric care environments, nurses have a chance to know their patients and their families. In long-term care facilities, they may care for the same person for years. The more familiar you are with a patient, the easier the job gets. Older people tend to have routines. When you get to know the way they like to do things, you can give them better care. For example, a patient may enjoy the bingo game that happens every morning at 10. That same person may have early signs of dementia and be forgetful. You can be helpful by bringing their morning pills and helping them get dressed at 9:30.

Geriatric patients are usually happy to see you. They see you more than they see their own family, and you are the one they depend on to keep them going. Seeing your smile as you enter the room is often the highlight of their day. Your warmth and empathy will often be rewarded with big hugs because older people tend to be more willing to show their gratitude. They appreciate your hard work and they do not mind telling you so!

Geriatric nurses know something most people do not – elderly people are great to be around. They have a ton of life experience and many stories to tell. The opportunity to learn from geriatric patients is one of the benefits nurses enjoy the most. Older people have a wealth of knowledge to share and time to do just that.

UNATTRACTIVE ASPECTS

GERIATRIC NURSING CAN BE IMMENSELY rewarding, but it is also hard work. It is physically strenuous, requiring the ability to lift patients who do not have the strength to fully transport themselves to the bathroom or turn over so that they do not develop bed sores. Physical exertion also is required when helping patients with prescribed therapeutic exercise regimens.

This work can be emotionally tiring as well. Older patients do not recover as quickly as younger people. A geriatric nurse has to be patient, yet cheerful, while reassuring depressed and discouraged patients. There is also a higher rate of loss among elderly patients, whether through disease or natural causes. Geriatric nurses often become close to those they are caring for. Being there for a patient who is facing the end of life can be sad and stressful. Not everyone is able to take the emotional toll.

Geriatric nurses get into this specialty because they enjoy working with older people. Most patients are delightful, but others may be bitter and mean. It may not be their fault – mental health is an issue of aging. Whether they mean to be difficult or not, geriatric nurses sometimes find themselves chasing people down hallways, picking up plates of food that have been thrown to the floor, or even dodging punches. Family members can be difficult, too, especially when they are feeling guilty or are having trouble dealing with the changes in their loved ones.

The nursing shortage has created tremendous opportunities for new and experienced geriatric nurses. That same shortage often results in chronic understaffing, particularly in LTCs. That results in heavier workloads for those working there.

EDUCATION AND TRAINING

THE TRAINING FOR GERIATRIC NURSES starts with the same core education as all other nurses. However, while some nurses can start with an associate degree, geriatric nurses need to become licensed Registered Nurses (RN). That means they must complete a registered nursing program, typically at the bachelor's degree level. After earning a Bachelor of Science degree in nursing (BSN), they must obtain a registered nurse (RN) license.

BSN programs generally take four years to complete. Programs vary somewhat with different schools, but most include classroom studies in anatomy, physiology, medical terminology, microbiology, chemistry, nutrition, psychology, patient care, ethics, and other physical and behavioral sciences. Like most bachelor's degree programs, nursing programs usually include additional education in the liberal arts, communication, leadership, and critical thinking. All programs include supervised clinical experience in non-hospital settings and in on-site clinics, or through internships.

Some undergraduate degree programs offer courses in geriatric nursing, but these are brief and introductory. Aspiring geriatric nurses must first become RNs, then continue their studies in the field of geriatrics through experiential hospital programs or through graduate studies.

Graduate studies and fellowship opportunities can prepare nurses for careers beyond direct patient care. A master's degree or higher is often needed for administrative positions, geriatric research, consulting, and academic positions. The programs, often known as adult health nursing programs, usually take two or three years to complete. The common coursework includes advanced subjects like nursing research, elderly nursing problems, pharmacology, and pathophysiology. Graduates are eligible to pursue advanced credentials, such as adult nurse practitioner certification from the American Nurses Credentialing Center (ANCC) .

Geriatric nurses who want to get involved in clinical research can pursue a PhD in Geriatric Nursing. This program can be completed in three years. The subject matter is very focused on research, covering various relevant topics such as research methodology and medical ethics. Doctoral students must complete and defend an original dissertation with consultation from a faculty panel.

Geriatric Nursing Assistants

This path is for those who want to start a career in geriatrics as quickly as possible. Becoming a geriatric nursing assistant or aide requires the completion of a nursing assistant program in a community college or geriatric aide-training program through a vocational school. These are typically short-term certificate programs that require less than a year of study. Basic coursework includes classes in human anatomy, nutrition, and physiology. The programs are designed to prepare the graduate for certification exams to become a CNA (Certified Nursing Assistant).

It is common for new CNAs to receive on-the-job training under the supervision of RNs and experienced geriatric nursing assistants. Hospitals and long-term care facilities often have formal training programs that include classes in personal care, communications skills (designed specifically for communicating with geriatric patients and their families), and patients' rights.

Licenses and Certifications

All geriatric nurses start out as registered nurses. All states, the District of Columbia, and US territories, require registered nurses to have a nursing license. To become licensed, nurses must graduate from an approved nursing program and pass the National Council Licensure Examination (NCLEX-RN). Other requirements for licensing, such as passing a criminal background check, vary by state. Each state's board of nursing has its own specific requirements.

To practice nursing in the geriatric field requires additional certification. Eligibility starts with completing 200 hours or more of hands-on experience as a registered nurse working with elderly patients. They must also pass a secondary certification exam called the Gerontological Nursing Certification, which is offered through the American Nurses Credentialing Center.

Certification is also necessary to become a geriatric nursing assistant. Successful completion of a state-approved program involving at least 75 hours of training is needed to become eligible for CNA certification. The National Council of State Boards of Nursing (NCSBN) offers a list of state-approved training programs on their website. In some states, you may be able to earn additional certification as a Certified Medication Assistant in order to administer medications to patients.

EARNINGS

MOST NURSES ARE ATTRACTED TO THE PROFESSION for the work itself, but while compassion and purpose are rewarded on a personal level, money is important, too. Nurses overall earn a good living, but those with a specialty tend to do better than those who generalize. Geriatrics is a growing specialty that offers a range of opportunities to earn more than the average nurse. Depending on geographic location, experience, level of education, and work environment, wages for geriatric nurses can vary greatly. Overall, the average annual salary for a geriatric nurse is about $65,000. That is a few thousand dollars more each year than the average RN makes.

The Northeast is particularly generous to geriatric nurses. The average income in states like Connecticut, New York, and Massachusetts is well above $90,000. The highest paid geriatric nurses in the country are in Washington DC, where the average salary is nearly $100,000. More sparsely populated states like the Dakotas, Nevada, Utah, and Wyoming pay the least. The average in places like these is well below the national average, hovering around $60,000. The lowest of all is Hawaii where the average is only $50,000 while the cost of living is high.

Geriatric nurses can increase their salaries by pursuing continuing and graduate education. Geriatric nurses with master's or doctoral degrees are highly sought after and because there are not enough of them to meet the demand, employers offer significant pay increases. For example, a graduate degree can lead to a geriatric nurse practitioner job that pays two to three times what a regular geriatric nurse earns. Most nurses start working immediately after graduating from nursing school. Typically, they do not return to pursue higher education until they have been on the job a few years. Fortunately, this is made fairly easy by both employers and schools. The schedule of educational programs normally allows students to continue working. In many cases, employers cover all or part of the training costs.

Geriatric nursing salaries vary widely depending on the type of employer. For example, residential care facilities and nursing homes pay less than hospitals. Hospitals pay $70,000 to $80,000 for staff geriatric nurses, while long-term care facilities offer an average of only $60,000.

Those who earn the highest are on the road. Becoming a traveling geriatric nurse is a good way to increase compensations. Traveling nurses earn outstanding wages, far surpassing the average income for staff nurses. Since geriatric nurses are needed everywhere, a traveling nurse can pick and choose where to accept assignments. In addition to great pay, traveling nurses receive subsidized housing, travel allowance, 401(k) contributions, and free CEUs (Continuing Education Units). Overall, that adds up to $100,000 in compensation annually. In shortage areas, there are additional perks designed to entice prospective contractors, such as per-diem allowances and free housing.

OPPORTUNITIES

NURSES WITH EXPERTISE IN GERIATRIC CARE are very much in demand. This particular type of nursing will see a significant increase in the number of available jobs that is far greater than the average for all occupations. Estimates of the job growth rate over the next decade are be between 20 and 25 percent. For years there has been a shortage of nurses in general, but the problem is much worse in the field of geriatrics. Geriatric nurses are now one of the most sought after healthcare professionals across the country.

Job growth will continue to surge for one main reason: the population is aging. More than 78 million people make up the Baby Boomer generation, named for the flood of babies born between 1946 and 1964. People in this age group started crossing the threshold into their 60s just over a decade ago. In another five years, the entire group will be retirement age. As they get farther into the 65-plus category, chronic illnesses and complications of aging are going to drive them to need additional healthcare.

Simply put, older people usually have more medical issues than younger people. In fact, twice as many people over the age of 65 make at least 10 more trips to the doctor per year than the average for any other age group. With the 78 million elderly people in the Baby Boomer bracket, combined with another 10 million born before 1946, and the total is one quarter of the population that will be in need of extra care for age-related health problems. Is it any wonder there is such an urgent demand for geriatric nurses?

Nurses who understand the biological and psychological changes of aging, and possess the skills to deal with the complexities of geriatric health issues will find opportunities in a variety of healthcare facilities. Hospitals, which previously relied on general RNs to care for all patients including the elderly, increasingly prefer nurses who have some related work experience or certification in specialty areas. Geriatrics is one of those areas. As the population ages, the number of hospital visits increases exponentially. Already, one half of all hospital admissions are for people who are 65 or older. Yet just one percent of nurses are trained to work in geriatric nursing. That makes for a wide-open field for newly certified geriatric nurses, particularly those who are bilingual in English and Spanish.

Opportunities are not limited to the hospital environment. There are numerous other eldercare providers that also need geriatric nurses to manage patients and residents. Some are specialty facilities and some are more general. For example, there are specialized rehabilitation centers dedicated to helping older people recover from injuries sustained from falls or other accidents. There are age-related differences and limitations associated with broken bones. If not treated appropriately, a broken bone can be fatal. Therefore, rehab nurses with geriatric skills are highly valued. Employers that are more general include places where there are large populations of elderly people, such as retirement communities and senior centers.

The largest traditional employer is the long-term care facility, also known as a nursing home. There are nearly 16,000 of these facilities in the US providing (licensed) beds to roughly two million elderly people. Long-term care facilities are notoriously understaffed. They have long struggled to attract enough certified geriatric nurses and often fill in the gaps with geriatric nursing assistants. Clearly, there is a wealth of opportunities for both.

There has been a growing trend toward keeping aging

people in their homes as long as possible. This has created the booming industry of home care services. Geriatric nurses in this arena work for agencies that assign them to a certain number of patients that they will visit in their homes each day. Opportunities also exist to advance in the career by earning certification as a geriatric care manager. Geriatric care managers have the choice of working with existing home health agencies or opening their own consultancies.

In between home care and long-term care is the assisted living facility. These facilities are designed to provide a homelike atmosphere for older people who are not able to live in their own home, but do not need the constant medical services of a nursing home. Assisted living facilities need geriatric nurses to help residents prevent or avoid infections and mishaps.

Hospice care provides end-of-life care, in the home or in a special facility. Geriatric nurses are the best-suited healthcare professionals to work with patients facing terminal illness and provide emotional support for their families. Opportunities abound for those special nurses with the appropriate education, experience, and understanding in this final stage of healthcare.

GETTING STARTED

THE NEED FOR GERIATRIC NURSES HAS never been greater. Once you have your training and get your nursing license, you can rest assured that there will be a job waiting for you. You may even receive multiple offers. To make sure you can land the job you want, there are things you can do to stand out in the field of candidates.

Expand your résumé with as much hands-on experience

as you can. While in school, participate in internships. If there are not any internships that specifically place you in geriatrics, get involved anyway. Any kind of nursing or healthcare experience will be considered a plus. In addition, you can get experience by volunteering. Nursing homes and assisted living centers are always in need of help – especially if you have some nursing education under your belt. All of this experience will demonstrate to potential employers that you understand what the work entails and have acquired the skills necessary to provide good geriatric care.

While getting experience through internships, volunteer positions, or part-time jobs, you should be building a network of contacts. Networking is very important in the nursing profession. Though there are many ways to find job openings, most nurses use their contacts to find the best jobs. Your network can start with supervisors and professors, but do not stop there. Join professional nursing associations and attend their conferences. Meet recruiters at career expos, join students groups in nursing school, and participate in work-study programs in local hospitals. In every situation that puts you in contact with potential employers, go out of your way to make your ambitions known and keep in touch.

Check in with your college career center. You will find job postings and notices of job fairs and upcoming visits from recruiters. There are also numerous other benefits such as help with writing résumés and opportunities to practice interviewing skills. You would be wise to take advantage of everything the career center has to offer.

Geriatric nursing jobs can be found online. Focus on the many sites devoted to the nursing field, such as NursingJobs.com and NurseRecruiter.com. Professional nursing associations also post jobs on their websites. You do not have to wait to see a job opening in a help wanted ad. If you know where you want to work, contact the potential employer directly. If you have someone in your network who can give you an introduction, that would be ideal. But if not, do not hesitate to introduce yourself.

Look beyond the obvious to find more opportunities. There are more possible work settings than you might imagine. It seems logical that geriatric nurses would work in hospitals, but that is only one environment among many that could use your skills. You could work for a community health center, a resort, a nonprofit health organization, or a retirement center. Also look outside your geographic area. In some locations around the country, the need for geriatric nurses is critical. Where that is the case, you can expect little competition.

Would you like to be paid while seeing the country? Consider becoming a traveling nurse. There are traveling nurses everywhere, and it is fast becoming a favorite mode of employment for employers and nurses alike. Traveling nurses are placed by agencies that specialize in per diem contracts. Tip: Sign up with more than one agency to ensure you always have multiple options to choose from. Contracts typically last two to three months, and you will be paid more than permanent staff nurses. In addition to good pay and the freedom to stay as busy (or not) as you want, you will have the opportunity to see how different employers operate.

ASSOCIATIONS

■ **Aging Life Care Association**
http://www.aginglifecare.org

■ **American Assisted Living Nurses Association (AALNA)**
www.alnursing.org

■ **American Geriatrics Society (AGS)**
https://www.americangeriatrics.org

■ **American Society on Aging (ASA)**
www.asaging.org

■ **Association for Career and Technical Education**
www.acteonline.org

■ **Gerontological Advanced Practice Nurses Association (GAPNA)**
https://www.gapna.org

■ **National Association of Professional Geriatric Care Managers (NAPGCM)**
http://www.aginglifecare.org

PERIODICAL

■ **Geriatric Nursing Journal**
www.gnjournal.com

WEBSITES

■ **American Nurses Credentialing Center (ANCC)**
http://www.nursecredentialing.org
/GerontologicalNursing

■ The Hartford Institute for Geriatric Nursing
https://hign.org

■ HOSA-Future Health Professionals
hosa.org

■ The National Council of State Boards of Nursing
(NCSBN)
https://www.ncsbn.org

■ Nurse.com Geriatric Jobs
https://www.nurse.com/jobs/browse/geriatrics